THE POWER OF THE PAUSE

PAUSE

CAROLINE TRICKEY

THE POWER OF THE PAUSE

Foreword

A Brief Pause Before the Book About Pauses

(IDEALLY READ IN A DRESSING GOWN YOU DEFINITELY DIDN'T MEAN TO WEAR ALL DAY.)

Right. Stop. Just... stop.

Before you gallop headlong into this book like it's the magical fix for all your life's chaos (spoiler: it's not), allow me a brief preamble.

This is not a diet book.

It will not teach you to chew your way to salvation through chia seeds and quiet desperation.
It won't ask you to blend kale into a joyless green sludge and call it wellness.
And there are precisely zero recipes for protein balls. You're welcome.

This is a book about pausing.

Not the monk-on-a-mountain kind of pause.
Not the one where you sip herbal tea, whisper affirmations and reconnect with your inner six-year-old.
Just the everyday, gloriously human-as-hell kind.

The kind you take mid-scroll, mid-binge, mid-overthinking-your-entire-existence, where you stop just long enough to ask:
"Wait... what am I actually doing?"

See, we've been taught to hustle, strive, achieve, consume — preferably all at once and with a mild undercurrent of anxiety.

Pausing, by contrast, looks suspicious. It's awkward. It's unproductive.
It doesn't earn points, likes or steps.
But that's precisely why it matters.

A pause is a tiny rebellion.
A moment of radical awareness in a world that wants you asleep at the wheel — as long as you're still buying stuff.

It's where you notice your life.
Your habits.
Your thoughts.
Yourself.

So no, this isn't a book about fixing you.
It's a reminder that you were never broken.
You've just been too bloody busy to notice.

Now, take a breath.
Not because it's spiritual.
Because it's *useful*.

Then let's get on with it.

Contents

Introduction

The Fast-Food Life & The Case for Slowing Down

IN WHICH WE DISCOVER THAT YOUR MOUTH ISN'T A RUBBISH CHUTE, YOUR BODY IS NOT AN UBER EATS DROP ZONE AND SLOWING DOWN MIGHT JUST BE THE SECRET TO FEELING SANE AROUND FOOD.

Picture this: you're halfway through a packet of barbecue rice crackers you didn't even remember opening. You blink. Your fingers are dusty, your brain is foggy and there's a vague sense of shame you'll later misdiagnose as gluten intolerance.

Welcome to modern eating.

We live in a world where food is abundant, attention is extinct and the only thing slower than our Wi-Fi is our capacity to pause before inhaling a muffin the size of a toddler's head. We're distracted, disjointed and darting from screen to screen like confused meerkats, wondering why we always feel just a little bit... meh.

And don't get me wrong, this isn't some smug kale smoothie monologue. I'm not here to tell you that enlightenment lies in sipping bone broth while staring at a sunset in child's pose. I'm here to point out something far simpler. Something you already know. Something so wildly obvious that it often escapes us entirely:

You're not actually tasting your life.
You're rushing through it. And food — that glorious, sensual, life-sustaining miracle — has become nothing more than background noise in the chaos.

You're eating while scrolling.
You're chewing while typing.
You're snacking while fighting with someone on the internet about whether almond milk is going to destroy the planet.

And at some point along the way, we stopped noticing what we're eating, why we're eating or whether we're even *hungry* in the first place. Our bodies — bless 'em — are whispering quiet truths like *"hey mate, that's enough"* or *"just checking in, could we maybe have a vegetable soon?"* and we're replying with... Doritos. And TikTok.

So what's going on? Why are we, as a species that evolved through foraging, hunting and feasting with family, now eating protein bars alone in traffic like confused raccoons?

The answer is tragically simple: **we've forgotten to pause.**

Not in the grand, spiritual, go-on-a-yoga-retreat-in-Bali way. I mean literally. Physically. Briefly.

We've forgotten to stop.

We're living in what I call the **Fast-Food Mindset**:

- If it's not instant, it's not worth it.
- If I feel something uncomfortable, I must fix it immediately.
- If there's food nearby, I may as well eat it.
- If I don't clean the plate, Greta will be sad.

But here's the delicious irony: the thing that can *actually* shift your entire relationship with food, with your body, with your emotions... is **ridiculously small.** It's not a juice cleanse. It's not a 12-week programme involving burpees and kale enemas.

It's a pause.

A teeny, tiny, beautifully rebellious act of *not doing.*

The pause is where your power lives. It's the creaky space between impulse and action. The beat between thought and response. The moment where you can say, "Hang on — do I even want this Tim Tam or am I just trying to silence the existential dread of being overworked and under-napped?"

Because here's the truth you probably already suspect in your quinoa-sprinkled soul:

Most of the time, **you're not eating because you're hungry.**
You're eating because you're *tired.* Or *stressed.* Or *bored.* Or *lonely.* Or you just saw an ad for melted cheese and now you can't remember your middle name.

And that's not a flaw. That's not weakness. That's not "being bad" or "having no willpower." That's being **human in the 21st century.**
You've just got a pattern. And like any pattern — be it biting your nails or dating emotionally unavailable DJs — it can be paused, rewired and changed.

This book is not here to shame you. (Frankly, you've had enough of that from your inner critic, your PT and the diet industry.)
This book is here to give you the one thing they never talk about: **a different way in.**

Not through punishment, but through presence.
Not through restriction, but through reflection.
Not by cutting carbs, but by carving space.

Because that pause — that breath, that blink, that moment of "Huh?"
— is where you go from *reacting* to *responding*.
From *numbing* to *noticing*.
From *mindless munching* to *mindful munching* (which, let's be honest, still might include chips, but this time with dignity).

So, here's the invitation:

Slow down.
Take a breath.
Taste your damn food.

You're not a robot. You're not a failure. You're not a dumpster for left-over kids' lunches.

You're a gloriously complex, beautifully sensitive, slightly chaotic miracle of a human being — and you deserve more than a life lived on autopilot.

So let's pause.

Let's pay attention.

Let's change it all — one bite, one breath, one beautiful, rebellious pause at a time.

1

~~~~~~

Autopilot Eating — Why We Zone Out With Food

Or, "Why did I just eat three slices of banana bread and I'm not even sure I liked the first one?"

Let's begin with a familiar scene. You walk into the kitchen. You open the fridge. You stare blankly, as if the meaning of life might be hidden behind the pickles. Then you see the leftover lasagna. You weren't hungry five seconds ago, but somehow you're now holding a fork like it's a weapon of mass consumption and your brain has left the building.

You eat. Mechanically. Mindlessly. Mysteriously.

And then — poof! — it's gone.

The lasagna. The moment. The awareness.

And you're left wondering, "Did I even *taste* that?"

This, my friend, is **Autopilot Eating** — and you're not alone in this weird little trance we all seem to fall into like moths to a fluorescent light.

The Science Bit (Don't Worry, No Test Later)

Here's the thing: humans are creatures of habit. We love routines, shortcuts, patterns. Your brain is a beautifully lazy organ. It likes to conserve energy (unless it's 2am and it suddenly remembers that embarrassing thing you said in Year 9).

So it builds little loops. Routines. Muscle memory. **Habit circuits.**

And eating — that most basic of biological needs — gets roped into this loop very early on. We do it a lot. We do it everywhere. And eventually, it becomes so automatic that we can do it with our eyes closed, our brains switched off and both hands still replying to a work email.

It goes a little something like this:

- **Cue:** You see food (or think of food or pass a shop or smell toast).
- **Craving:** Your brain lights up like a slot machine: "Ooh! Pleasure coming!"
- **Routine:** Eat. Fast. Distracted. Possibly while also unloading the dishwasher.
- **Reward:** Tiny dopamine hit, followed by vague guilt, bloating or crumbs on your jumper.

This is the **habit loop**. It's like the backing track of your eating behaviour — and most of us don't even know it's playing. We just move through the motions, again and again, wondering why we never feel truly *satisfied*.

Distraction Culture: We're All Just Scrolling Zombies

And it's not just the habits. It's the context. The cultural soup we're all swimming in. The era of multitasking, micro-attention and constant bloody notifications.

We don't eat meals anymore. We eat *while*.

- While working.
- While driving.
- While watching Netflix's "Are you still watching?" judgement screen.
- While doom-scrolling Instagram accounts of people who apparently live in white linen clothing and eat chia pudding from coconut shells.

We're not present. We're not tuned in. We're consuming food the same way we consume content — fast, distracted and with a low-key sense of FOMO that maybe we should be eating something better, cooler or macro-balanced.

And ironically, the more we distract ourselves from the act of eating, the *more* we tend to eat. Because if your brain doesn't register the experience, it keeps shouting, "Oi! What was that? I missed it! Do it again!"

Hence: the mysterious disappearance of an entire bag of popcorn during what was supposed to be just a quick catch-your-breath break.

Emotional Numbing: When Food Is a Hug in Disguise

Let's go deeper. Because often, autopilot eating isn't just a harmless habit or a side effect of distraction. Sometimes, it's your body trying to *speak* and your brain throwing a sandwich at it to shut it up.

We eat to escape feelings.

I mean, *who doesn't?*

Food is comfort. Food is safe. Food doesn't judge you or ghost you or tell you you're being too sensitive.

When you're stressed, anxious, sad, bored, lonely — food shows up. It doesn't ask questions. It doesn't solve your problems either, but hey, at least it comes with salt and vinegar.

And here's where it gets sneaky: because it works. *Temporarily.* That cookie *does* make you feel better — for about six minutes. Then your brain's like, "Cool, we dodged that uncomfortable emotion. Let's never feel it again. Have another cookie."

Thus: the emotional numbing loop.

You feel something → You eat → You avoid → You repeat → You wonder why you still feel crap and also where all the cookies went.

It's not a character flaw. It's not emotional weakness. It's just a *pattern.*

And once you start seeing it clearly, you can change it. Which brings us to the punchline...

Change Doesn't Start with Willpower — It Starts with Awareness

This book isn't going to tell you to "just stop eating when you're full." That's like telling someone in a speeding car to "just stop" while they're still flying down the highway with no brakes and a goose in the passenger seat.

Willpower is overrated. It's the fitness tracker of the behaviour change world — it looks great for about a week, then it runs out of battery and ends up in a drawer next to your guilt and unused resistance bands.

The real magic? **Awareness.**

Change starts when you notice.
When you pause.
When you *feel* instead of flee.
When you go, "Oh, wow, I'm eating because I'm tired, not hungry." Or "I'm halfway through this burrito and I'm already done, but my mouth didn't get the memo."

That's the pause. The moment you shift from *autopilot* to *agency*. From *numbing* to *noticing*.

From "Ugh, I've got no self-control" to "Oh, I see what's going on here."

And that — *that* — is when the game changes.

Not because you forced it. But because you *woke up* to it.

So, now you know what you're working with: a brain that loves short-cuts, a world that worships distraction and a culture that equates hunger with failure and full with guilt.

But you've also got a secret weapon: awareness.

And that's what the next chapter is all about — learning to *pause*, to check in and to gently (but firmly) reclaim the wheel from the snack-craving autopilot gremlin inside your head.

Shall we?

2

❧

The Pause — Your Superpower in Disguise

Or, "How Five Seconds of Silence Can Save You From an Entire Family-Sized Bag of Twisties"

Let's start with a bold claim: **the pause is not just a moment. It's a bloody superpower.**

It may not sound as sexy as flying or invisibility or being able to cook rice without checking the packet 14 times, but when it comes to food, emotions, habits and that little thing called life — the pause is a game-changer. A quiet, sneaky, often-overlooked little Jedi mind trick that separates the women from the wild snack wolves.

So... What Actually *Is* the Pause?

The pause is that itty-bitty space between a trigger and your reaction.

Someone brings out cupcakes at work — **trigger.**
Your hand's halfway to the tray before your brain even checks in — **re-action.**

But right in the middle...Just before that fluffy cream cheese icing hits your fingers...
There's a gap. A fraction of a second. A single breath.

That is the pause.
And in that micro-moment lies your freedom.
Ooooh, deep.

It's the place where your inner grown-up gets a chance to whisper, "Do I really want this?"
Instead of letting your inner toddler scream, "CAKE IS HAPPINESS! EAT NOW OR DIE."

Why the Pause Works: Neuroscience Meets Nonsense

Let's nerd out for a second. Your brain has two main systems in this story:

- **The Limbic System** (a.k.a. your inner gremlin): it's fast, emotional, impulsive and very good at spotting danger or free samples.
- **The Prefrontal Cortex** (a.k.a. your wise inner Yoda): it's logical, thoughtful and capable of long-term decision-making... but it's a bit slow on the uptake.

When a craving hits or an emotion flares or a family member breathes too loudly, your limbic system leaps into action like a caffeinated meerkat. It wants relief and it wants it *now*. Food becomes the answer, the fix, the hero on a white chocolate steed.

But when you pause — just for 5 seconds — you give your prefrontal cortex a chance to *show up to the party*. And once it's in the room, the whole vibe changes.

Instead of reacting, you start **responding**.

You ask:

- Am I actually hungry?
- What am I feeling?
- Will this third lamington help or just make me need a nap?

And boom — you've interrupted the loop. You've gone from passenger to pilot. From "oops I did it again" to "actually... nah, I'm good."

Five Seconds That Rewire Your Brain (No Cape Required)

Here's the sexy science: studies in neuroscience show that **pausing activates the dorsolateral prefrontal cortex** — the bit of your brain responsible for self-control, planning and not throwing your phone across the room during a slow Zoom meeting.

It also helps **downregulate the amygdala** — your brain's fear-and-feeling centre, which is lovely and helpful in a bear attack, but slightly dramatic when your boss sends you a vaguely passive-aggressive email and you decide to eat your feelings via a block of Cadbury.

In short: the pause **turns down reactivity** and **turns up regulation**.

And while five seconds might sound laughably small, it's like the clutch in a car. It's the mechanism that lets you **shift gears**, rather than just accelerating straight into "stuff-your-face" mode.

You don't need to meditate for an hour or chant while holding a crystal (though you do you, babe). You just need to *breathe*. Notice. Check in.

And that check-in is *everything*.

From Autopilot to Awareness: The Magic of Mindful Interruptions

Let's say you're elbow-deep in a packet of chips. No judgement. We've all been there. Somewhere between chip 7 and chip 73, you pause. You look at your hand. You take a breath. You notice the taste. The crunch. The fact that you're not actually enjoying them anymore.

In that pause, you return to *presence*.
You reconnect to *choice*.
You reclaim *power*.

Because that's what the pause really is — it's **choice in disguise**.

And choice, my friend, is the gateway drug to freedom.

Without the pause, we eat out of habit, boredom, stress, peer pressure, proximity or because we've mistaken thirst for a deep spiritual calling to eat toast.

With the pause, we eat because we *choose to* — not because we have to.

But Isn't This Just... Mindfulness?

Yes. Sort of. But let's be honest, "mindfulness" has been stuck to so many things it's practically lost all meaning. Mindful emails. Mindful spreadsheets. Mindful washing-up (which is just regular washing-up but while hating it slightly less).

What we're talking about here is **practical mindfulness**. Everyday, bite-sized, no-nonsense noticing. No robes required.

It's noticing when you're about to eat.
Noticing how you feel.
Noticing what you actually want.

And giving yourself the radical, revolutionary permission to *pause and decide.*

Try This (Without Rolling Your Eyes)

Next time you're about to eat — anything — try this:

1. **Pause** before the first bite.
2. Take a breath. Like, an actual inhale-exhale situation.
3. Ask, *"What do I need right now?"*

Then — and this bit is key — *listen.*
If the answer is "I'm bloody hungry," then eat! Gloriously!
If the answer is "I'm actually just tired and looking for a distraction," then... maybe you nap, walk or scream into a pillow instead. Who knows? Life's a buffet.

But either way, you've disrupted the loop.

You've broken the trance.
You've gone from autopilot to author.
And you've started reprogramming your brain in the tiniest — but mightiest — of ways.

So there you have it.
A superpower that doesn't require a cape, a six-week course or a Pinterest-worthy smoothie bowl.
Just five seconds.
A breath.
And a little bit of "Hmm... what's actually going on here?"

In the next chapter, we're zooming in on something deceptively simple: actually tasting your food.

Not in a "chew each almond thirty-two times" kind of way.

In a "be in the room with your mouth" kind of way.

Because mindfulness isn't just some woo-woo wellness trend. It's the secret weapon against fridge raids, distracted dinners and wondering where your lunch went.

Spoiler alert: you don't need wind chimes, crystals or a guy named Sage.

Just your senses.

Because when you notice the bite,
You notice *you're* the one taking it.

And that tiny shift?
It changes everything.

3

The Art of the Mindful Bite

(Or: How to Actually Taste Your Food Without Joining a Cult)

L et's be honest.

You've probably heard about mindful eating before — and promptly imagined some guy named Sage whispering affirmations to his lentils.

And look, good on Sage. But if your reaction was, "I don't have time to chew each almond thirty-two times while contemplating my inner child and the almond's tragic journey from tree to trail mix" — you're not alone.

And you're right.

Because mindful eating isn't about being precious or weird or chewing in a way that would get you politely uninvited from future dinner parties.

It's about one thing: **noticing that you're eating**.

That's it.

That's the whole gig.

Mindfulness = awareness.
Mindless = shovelling food into your face like a raccoon in a skip bin.

And let's face it — we've all been there. Eating an entire bag of potato chips while watching Netflix, only to look down and realise the bag is empty… and you have zero recollection of chewing. Just salty finger-tips and existential questions.

So. Let's bring you back.
To the bite.
To the taste.
To the bloody point of eating: **pleasure, nourishment and not turning into a hangry gremlin.**

Sane, Smart Ways to Eat Like You're Actually in the Room

Because you've got a palate, not just a pie hole — and meals taste way better when your brain's invited to the party.

Let's make eating feel intentional, not accidental.

1. The First Bite Rule

The first bite is the Beyoncé of the meal.

It's the one your brain pays the most attention to. It's the peak of the experience. The applause moment.

So give it a second.

Pause.

Taste it like it matters — because it does. That first bite delivers the biggest hit of satisfaction. Nail it and you might find you don't need the entire cake to feel content. Half the cake will do.

(Just kidding. Sort of.)

2. Cutlery Exists for a Reason

Sometimes, the simple act of putting your fork down between bites is enough to shift you from hoover mode to human mode.

When you don't eat like you're trying to win a timed event, magical things happen:

You notice when you're full.

You actually taste your food.

You avoid that tragic moment where you look down and think, "Where the hell did it all go?"

3. Make It a Full Sensory Party

You don't need to hold a strawberry and whisper sweet nothings to it.

But noticing colour, smell, texture and flavour? That's a gateway drug to satisfaction.

And satisfaction = less likelihood of going back for round two, three or "oops I finished the whole box."

So next time you're eating, try this:

"What does this feel like in my mouth? Crunchy? Creamy? Explosively sweet like a mango doing a happy dance?"

Bring in the senses. Let your mouth, nose, eyes, ears and tongue get in on the action and fully experience the food. And don't give air time to any mental noise trying to hijack the moment — no guilt, no judgement, just you and your food.

Mindfulness: It's Not Just for Monks and People Who Own Wind Chimes

You don't need to be "zen" to eat mindfully.

You just need to be not asleep at the mental wheel.

Try this little experiment:

Next time you eat — a snack, a meal, even just a bite — do it without your phone, your laptop or your "I'm just checking one email" brain.

Just eat.

Notice. Chew. Taste. Swallow. Breathe.

Boom. You're officially doing mindfulness. No crystals required.

And you know what else?

It changes the game.

Suddenly, one piece of dark chocolate becomes deeply satisfying, not a warm-up act for demolishing the block. A slice of pizza tastes like a slice of pizza, not "that thing I inhaled while watching a murder documentary and checking notifications."

But What If I Forget and Eat Like a Goblin Again?

Ah yes — the inevitable moment:
"I just ate the whole thing... standing up... in the fridge light."

Here's the deal: you're human. Not a monk. Not a robot. You will forget. You will hoover sometimes. It's OK.

The goal isn't to be perfect. It's to be aware — **more often**.

Every mindful bite is a win.
A small act of rebellion against autopilot eating.
A little gift to your body and your sanity.

It's the difference between eating a croissant and experiencing a croissant. (Flaky, buttery, serious yumminess.)

And trust me — food tastes better when you're actually there for it.

So yes—mindful bites matter.
They bring you back into the moment. Into your body. Into choice.

But what about the moments when you *don't* pause?
When the bite's already halfway to your mouth and a quiet little thought slips in—
"Who cares?"

And you believe it, without question.

Next chapter, we're calling that voice out.
Because not every thought deserves your trust.
And just because your brain says it, doesn't mean it's true.

4

⚜

"Who Cares"

(And Other Lies We Tell Ourselves While Holding a Biscuit)

There's a moment—microscopic, silent, slippery—When you *know* you're about to do the thing. You feel the fork lift, the fridge open, the packet rustle...

And a thought bubbles up, wrapped in logic-flavoured fairy floss:

"Who cares?"

It's such a tidy little sentence,
Perfectly polished like a turd in a tuxedo.
And it sounds *so true*.
So... *reasonable*.
So... defeatishly freeing.

Because it's not *you*, right? It's the urge!
The craving! The day!
The government!

Your boss!
Your mother!
The *vibe*!

But what you're really up against...
Is a **habitual sentence**.
A recycled, rerun thought pattern
That your brain's been playing like a 90s sitcom
Just before dinner since you were 14.

Excuses.
Just *sentences*. Not truth.
Just lizard-brain linguistics designed
To get you to the dopamine as quickly as possible.
They're not logic. They're just... efficiency.

"Stuff it, I deserve this."
"It's Friday."
"It's raining."
"I'm tired."
"I'm bored."
"I'm breathing."

Every excuse is just your lower brain
Putting on a tiny monocle,
Pretending to be wise and worldly,
While actually being a toddler in the lolly aisle,
Screaming, "Now!"

And your prefrontal cortex—the adult in the room—
Wants to say,
"Mate, we've had this conversation 37 times. We CARE."
But the toddler is LOUD.

And you're tired.
And, honestly, *who cares?*

You do.

Of course you care.
You're just not always able to *access* the part of you that cares
In that high-stakes moment
Between craving and cookie.

And so, instead of facing the discomfort of saying no,
You opt for the *false comfort* of giving in.

You think the urge is what's strong.
But it's not.
It's the excuse.
The sentence.
The pre-packaged permission slip your brain keeps handing you.
Signed in ink and guilt.

And here's the kicker:
You don't have to *argue* with it.
You don't have to *wrestle* it.

You just have to pause.
And in that pause, you'll see it for what it is:

Neural graffiti.
Cognitive spam.
Brain burps.

And you say,
"Oh, there's that one again. 'Who cares?'
Cute. I do, actually."
And then—brace yourself—

You say **no**.
Or maybe **not now**.
Or even just **...wait a minute.**

Yes, it'll feel uncomfortable.
Yes, your toddler-brain will throw a tantrum.
But here's the thing:

The price of that discomfort?
It's the currency of becoming the version of you
Who knows how to steer the car
Instead of handing the keys to your inner goblin.

The more you face the feeling,
The less it will knock you down.
The more you sit in the discomfort,
The more you realise—it's not even that bad.
It's just unfamiliar.
Not fatal.
Just *practice*.

And over time,
That voice in your head that says,
"Who cares?"
Will sound a little more sheepish.
A little more obvious.
A little more... full of shit.

And your answer will be clear.

"I do. That's who."

So now you've seen it—how that one sneaky thought can hijack your logic and fast-track you to the biscuit tin.

But it's not just that thought.

It's the whole *loop* it triggers.

Next up, we're pulling back the curtain on the full production: the cues, the cravings, the routines, the rewards.

Because the moment you start seeing the loop, you can stop being stuck in it.

Let's go.

5

Interrupting the Loop

Using Pauses to Break Old Patterns

*OR, "HOW TO STOP EATING LIKE IT'S A COM-
PETITIVE SPORT AND YOU'RE THE UNDIS-
PUTED CHAMPION OF NUMBING"*

Let's talk about loops.

Not the reruns of rubbish TV shows you watch just to feel slightly less awful about your life choices.
Not those endless social media scroll-loops where you lose 45 minutes and come out the other end questioning your own thumbs.

No, I'm talking about **habit loops** — those sneaky little neural reruns that make you eat like you're possessed by the ghost of Hungry You Past, Present and Future.

You know the ones.

- You feel stressed → eat chocolate.
- You're bored → open the fridge.
- You walk into a cinema → you're instantly holding popcorn and you have no idea how it got there.

That's a habit loop, baby.
Cue dramatic music...*Dun dun duuuuun.*

What is a Habit Loop?

A habit loop is essentially your brain doing a weird version of Groundhog Day. It's made up of four parts:

1. **Cue** – something happens.
2. **Craving** – you want to feel better.
3. **Routine** – you do something.
4. **Reward** – you feel something (usually better, briefly, before regret strolls in wearing pyjamas and holding a spoon).

Your brain loves this. It's efficient. Familiar. Like a shortcut through a dodgy alley — quick, yes, but also littered with weird smells and emotional potholes.

And here's the kicker: every time you repeat the loop, it gets stronger. Like a groove in a vinyl record.
Or that one stubborn wheel on a shopping trolley that insists on veering left, no matter how hard you try to steer it straight ahead.

Why We Loop (Even When We Know Better)

Let me make this painfully clear: **Nothing's wrong with you** for eating the leftover cake at 10:43pm—even if you're not hungry and the cake is a bit dry.

You're just looping.

You've taught your brain — repeatedly — that certain cues (like stress, tiredness, loneliness or celebratory vibes) = food = momentary relief.

So your brain, being helpful but dim, says, *"Oh great! We're stressed again! I know what to do! Deploy the emergency protocol: inhale the pantry, interrogate the freezer and if things get really dire… there's always the baking chocolate."*

This is why **willpower doesn't work long-term**.
Because your habit loop is faster than your logic.
It's like trying to win a fencing match with a cooked spaghetti noodle.

So what does work?

Say it with me now...

The Pause: Your Habit Loop Hacker

Remember in the last chapter when we lovingly worshipped the pause as your inner superhero? Well now we're weaponising it.

Not in a scary, Marvel-universe way. More like a laser pointer for your awareness.

See, **the pause is how you interrupt the loop before it becomes a re-play**.

It slips in between the cue and the routine.
It lets you *notice* the urge before you act on it.
It gives your brain a moment to ask, *"Wait... do I really want this? Or am I just emotionally constipated?"*

That's the magic.

You're not fighting the urge.
You're just observing it.

Like watching a toddler throw a tantrum in the supermarket and going, *"Wow. That's intense. Thankfully not my small, sticky problem."*

Try This: The 3-Step Loop Interruptor

You don't need incense.
You don't need to be wearing linen.
You just need this:

1. Notice & Name

Notice the Cue
You feel something: stressed, tired, lonely, elated, anxious, awkward at a party where everyone knows someone but the only thing familiar to you is the cheese platter.

Name it. *"Oh look, there's frustration. Classic."*

2. Pause Before the Routine
Take 5 seconds. Breathe. Let the urge to raid the fridge just… exist, without acting on it.
Feel the squirm. The tension. The itchy, twitchy need for relief.
This is the gold. **This is where the loop loses power.**

3. Choose a New Response
Ask:
   "What do I *really* need?"
   "What would Future Me be proud of?"
   "Is this hunger… or just a vibe?"
And then… you choose. Maybe you eat. Maybe you don't. But you're back in the driver's seat and that's where change begins.

But What If I Still Eat the Cake?

Good. You're human.

The goal isn't to pause and become a floating monk who survives on filtered thoughts and green tea.
The goal is to pause and become *aware*. To *choose*. To say, *"Yep, I'm eating this cake and I'm gonna enjoy the crap out of it."*

Because that's what interrupts the shame spiral.

You didn't fail. You *chose*.
You didn't react. You *responded*.
And every time you do that — even imperfectly — you're rewiring the loop.

And over time, those new grooves become your new normal.

Less reacting. More choosing.
Less "I don't know what happened." More "I saw it, I paused and I did what felt right."

The Slow Burn Wins

Let's be honest. This work - It's not fast.
You won't be a Zen master by next Thursday.
There's no six-day miracle that will erase decades of habits with green smoothies and good intentions.

But it *is* possible.
One pause at a time.

Interrupting the loop isn't about never eating emotionally again.
It's about knowing *when you are* and deciding if that's what you need.
It's about building trust with yourself, tiny choice by tiny choice.

It's about showing your brain that you're not at the mercy of every whim, urge or leftover trifle.

You've got a brain.
You've got awareness.
And you've got a superpower that fits in your pocket and takes five seconds.

Not bad, hey?

Next up? We're diving into cravings: what they *really* are, why they feel like hostage negotiations and how to surf them like a boss instead of drowning in them like a soggy chip in the deep fryer of doom.

Bring your inner scientist. And a snack. You'll want both.

6

⊚≋

Cravings, Hijacks & Emotional Hurricane

Or, "Why You're Not Weak, You're Wired That Way — Now Let's Hack It"

L et's set the scene.

You're standing in the kitchen. Again.

You've opened the fridge 14 times in the last 7 minutes. That poor fridge light is starting to get performance anxiety.

You're not hungry. You *know* you're not hungry.

You even said, *"I'm just going to look."*

Liar.

You spot the cheese. The leftover Thai. That one sad chocolate biscuit hanging on for dear life in a half-crumpled packet.

And boom — the mental wrestling match begins.

"Should I?"
"But I'm not hungry."
"But I want it."
"But I'm trying to be good."
"But it's been a day, Cheryl."

Welcome to the neon-lit circus of cravings, emotional hijacks and "what the hell just happened?" food decisions.

Pull up a chair, my fellow human. You're not fundamentally flawed. You're just brilliantly, biologically wired — with a few default settings that need a gentle, loving hack.

Let's do some neurological spelunking, shall we?

Cravings Aren't the Enemy — They're Just Misunderstood Performance Artists

Cravings get a bad rap.

We paint them as villains — shadowy, seductive, sent to sabotage your progress with the stealth of a ninja and the persistence of a toddler on red cordial.

But here's the backstage truth: cravings aren't evil.

They're just internal messengers dressed in emotionally confusing drag.

A craving is your nervous system's equivalent of a *ding!*
"Hey! Something's going on! Pay attention!"

They might be saying:

- "I'm tired and need energy, stat!"
- "I'm stressed and need soothing or possibly a therapist."
- "I'm bored and need something more stimulating than this f***ing spreadsheet."

Cravings are like emotional flare guns — *not* moral failings.
So the aim isn't to slap them away.

It's to *listen.*
Decode.
Maybe even thank them — and then *not* eat the entire pantry.

What's Actually Going on Upstairs (aka Science Time with Swear Words)

Let me introduce your amygdala — a delightful little almond-shaped nugget in your brain whose main job is to scan for threats.

And by "threats," I mean *feelings.*

Frustration? Threat.
Sadness? Threat.
Someone telling you in a patronising tone to *just calm down?* Major f*ing threat.

When your amygdala senses a storm brewing (even an emotional one), it hijacks the controls like a raccoon hopped up on Red Bull.

It boots your rational brain — the prefrontal cortex, our thoughtful CEO — straight off the stage.

Now the toddler's driving.

What happens next?
Impulse.
Craving.
Reaction.

Chips. Wine. Bread. Cheese. *Whatever combo your brain has decided is your quickest ticket to "make the feeling go away."*

This is *not* a failure of willpower.

It's a feature.
Your brain thinks it's protecting you — with snacks.

Which is honestly very sweet... and very unhelpful.

Cravings Are Waves — Not Tsunamis (Unless You Panic)

Let's talk cravings.
You know, that electrifying moment when your brain goes,
"EAT THE THING. DO IT NOW. OR THE WORLD ENDS."
(Which is dramatic, considering it's just a bloody muffin.)

But here's the inconvenient truth — the kind they don't stitch on tea towels or put in Instagram ads for 'clean' protein balls:
Cravings rise.
They peak.
And — plot twist — they pass.

They're waves.
Not serene, poetic waves that gently lap the shore while some ukulele plays in the background.
No no.
We're talking proper Aussie surf — the kind that smacks you square in the face, knocks your sunnies off and sends your dignity to Narnia.

Still — they're just waves.
Not tsunamis.
Unless you panic.
Then you're just flailing around, trying to plug a leaky boat with a Tim Tam.

But here's where it gets *very* cool (and a little Matrix-y):
If you can resist the urge to bolt, binge or bash yourself over the head with guilt,
they pass.
You ride the wave.
You don't drown in it.

Enter: **The Pause.**
Yes, her again. I know. She's the star of this show.

The queen of mindfulness.
The Gandalf of snack-time decisions.
She stands there in your brain whispering,

"You've got this. You can handle it."

But wait — it gets even better.
Let's introduce her enigmatic cousin.
She's got tattoos, does breathwork, listens to lo-fi beats in candlelight and once spent six weeks in a yurt just to "feel her feelings."

Urge Surfing: Ride the Craving, Don't Let It Ride You
This is next-level pause.
It's not "Hmm, maybe not the biscuit."
It's: **"Ah, I see you craving, you seductive bastard. Let's tango."**

Urge surfing is when you

- Notice the urge

- Nod at it like an old mate at the pub
- And then... just **be** with it

No drama. No wrestling. No peanut butter spoon sword fights.
Just awareness, baby.
It's mindfulness, turned up to 11.

A regular pause is like slamming the brakes.
Urge surfing...That's climbing onto your emotional surfboard, flexing your inner thighs and going
"Wheeeee! Let's feel some sh*t today!"

And here's the kicker:
The more you do it,
The stronger you get.
Emotionally. Neurologically. Existentially.
Like yoga for your dopamine pathways.

Soon, you're not just allowing cravings.
You're understanding yourself.

You're not avoiding food.
You're choosing.

You're not reacting.
You're *responding*.

And my friend, that's the magic.
Not in the calories or the macros or the latest almond milk made of moon dust.
But in the moment you say,
"I see the wave. I feel the wave. And I'm still here."

It builds emotional muscle. And with time, it rewires not just how you deal with cravings...

But how you deal with *you*.

Here's How to Urge Surf Like a Legend (Without Falling Into the Biscuit Tin):

1. Notice & Name It
"Oh hey there old friend."
Name it. "My old friend craving."
Naming moves you out of autopilot and into awareness — the first step to changing anything.

2. Feel It (Yes, the Uncomfortable Bit)
Cravings usually show up somewhere in the body.
A pull in your gut. A tightness in your chest. That weird feeling in your jaw that says, "Find chocolate, now."

Don't run. Don't fix.
Just breathe and notice.

3. Describe the Sensation (Optional, But Powerful)
Ask:

- Where do I feel this?
- What does it feel like — tight, buzzy, heavy?
- Does it move?
- Can I breathe into it?

You're not analysing. You're observing. Like David Attenborough, but inside your own body.

4. Surf It
Watch it rise.
Stay with it.
Notice it peak.

And — here's the magic — let it pass.

The craving might say, "EAT THE BISCUIT NOW OR WE DIE."
You acknowledge it. You breathe. You stay. You don't flinch.

And after 5, maybe 10 minutes?
The wave rolls back.
You're still standing.
The biscuit is still in the pantry.
You win.

5. Choose What Comes Next (Consciously)
Maybe you still want the thing. Maybe you don't.
The difference?
You're now choosing from awareness, not reactivity.

You didn't suppress.
You didn't give in.
You *surfed*.
Cue the internal slow clap.

Let's Debunk the Myth of "Control" (aka Willpower is a Wanker)

Here's something no one on Instagram with a 12-pack and a protein shake obsession will tell you:

"Controlling cravings" is a toxic fairytale.

White-knuckling your way through life — dodging joy, fearing food, avoiding cake like it's cocaine — that's not control. That's self-inflicted purgatory.

What you *actually* want is something way better:

Awareness + Response.

Noticing the urge.
Allowing the feeling.
Choosing your next move — with clarity and kindness.

That's not weakness.
That's bloody power.

Final Thought (Before You Headbutt the Fridge Again)

Cravings are not proof that you've failed.
They're proof that you *feel*.

Learning to sit with those feelings — awkwardly, imperfectly, beautifully — is how you build a relationship with food that doesn't come with shame, regret or an existential crisis mid-bite.

This isn't about being perfect.
It's about being powerful.

The kind of power that pauses.
That listens.
That responds — not reacts.

The kind of power that can look at a craving, wink and say:
"I see you. But I'm not your puppet anymore."

Now that's sexy.

Next up?

So... cravings. Not weakness. Not sabotage. Just misunderstood brain flares trying to help in the only way they know how.

And while it's tempting to slam the door on them, what if — hear me out — they're actually offering you something?

Insight. *Oooh deep.*

Next chapter, we're flipping the script.

Because cravings aren't a problem to solve.

They're a message.

A gift.

And it's time to start listening.

7

The Gift Of Cravings

A Musical Monologue

Ladies and gentlemen, gather 'round for a tale,
Of cravings and habits that often derail.
A journey through urges, both subtle and loud,
In the theatre of minds where desires are proud.

The Craving's Call

In the quiet of evening, when the world slows its pace,
A whisper emerges, a familiar face.
It's the craving, the yearning, the siren's sweet song,
Promising comfort where things have gone wrong.

But what if, dear friends, we paused to inquire,
What lies at the heart of this burning desire?
Is it hunger or habit or something more deep?
A need for connection or a longing to weep?

The Gift of Cravings

Oh, the gift of cravings, a message in disguise,
Not a foe to battle, but a signal to the wise.
They beckon us inward, to feelings we evade,
Inviting introspection, where true change is made.

The Mismatch of Needs

We reach for the chocolate, the wine or the cake,
Seeking solace in sweets for the heartache's sake.
But often, these treats are a mismatched reply,
To needs unacknowledged, to truths we deny.

Perhaps it's not sugar our bodies require,
But rest for the weary or warmth by the fire.
A moment of silence, a breath to be still,
To sit with our thoughts, to feel what we feel.

The Neutral Ground

Cravings aren't villains, nor virtues to praise,
They're neutral, they're natural, in so many ways.
It's the stories we tell them, the power we assign,
That shapes our reactions, our choices, our line.

So next time a craving comes knocking your way,
Don't shun it, don't shame it, don't wish it away.
Invite it to tea, ask what it's about,
Listen with kindness, dispelling the doubt.

The Gift of Cravings (Reprise)

Yes, the gift of cravings, a compass, a guide,
Pointing to places where feelings reside.
Not to be feared, but to be understood,
A path to self-awareness, to our greater good.

The Habitual Dance

"I'll be good tomorrow," we often proclaim,
As if virtue's a voucher we can easily claim.
But postponing our choices, deferring the now,
Keeps us tethered to habits we wish to disavow.

Change doesn't happen in some distant land,
It's forged in the moments where we take a stand.
To feel the discomfort, to sit with the urge,
To let the wave pass, to resist the surge.

Embracing the Craving

So here's to the cravings, the lessons they bring,
The songs of our psyche, the truths that they sing.
Embrace them, explore them, let them unfold,
For within them lies wisdom, more precious than gold.

Remember, the next time a craving whispers in your ear, don't just reach for the cookie jar.

Pause, listen and ask, "What is it you're truly telling me?"

Because sometimes, the sweetest gift is understanding ourselves a little better.

Curtain falls.

Next up? Chapter 8: *Emotional Eating — It's Not About the Food, But Let's Talk About It Anyway.*
Spoiler: You're not eating because you lack willpower or discipline. You're eating because you're trying to cope. And there is a better way.

Ready? Let's get into the messy middle.

8

⸎

Emotional Eating

It's Not About the Food, But Let's Talk About It Anyway

Let's be honest. If emotional eating were an Olympic sport, some of us would have gold medals, endorsement deals and a Wheaties box with our face on it.

We've all done it.

Eaten a packet of Tim Tams because we had "quite the day!"
Scoffed half a lasagne while binge-watching reality t.v.
Used Nutella like it was some kind of brown, hazelnut-scented emotional duct tape.

It's common. It's human. It's nothing to be ashamed of.

But — and it's a big but (and not just from the snacks) — if we don't understand *why* we emotionally eat, we'll keep doing it on autopilot. And that's where it becomes a problem, not just a coping strategy.

So today, my friends, we're taking off the shame-sweater and getting curious. Not judgy. Not "I'm such a failure." Just *curious*.

Because here's the thesis of this chapter, in bold font and full spotlight:

Emotional eating isn't about the food.
It's about what you're feeling... and what you don't want to feel.

Shall we begin?

Eating Feelings: The Less Romantic Sequel to "Eating, Pray, Love"

Let's set the scene again. You're in your kitchen (why is it always the kitchen?) with a spoon and a tub of ice cream. Or the couch. Or the car. Or crouched in the pantry like a snack-seeking gremlin.

And you're not hungry. You *know* you're not hungry.

So what are you?

Lonely?
Anxious?
Overwhelmed?
Bored enough to start reorganising your spice rack by chakra?

Emotional eating is what happens when food becomes therapy, entertainment, distraction or sedative. It's not about hunger — it's about *avoidance*.

You're not eating because you want to taste the creamy notes of camembert.
You're eating to avoid the uncomfortable feeling of being... well, *you*, in that moment.

And spoiler alert: everyone does this.
We all have our "thing" — food, wine, online shopping, obsessively

Googling symptoms until we convince ourselves we have three rare diseases and a vitamin B deficiency.

The key isn't to eliminate every emotional bite. The key is to understand what's behind it, so it's no longer in charge.

The Brain's Sneaky Little Shortcut:

Feel Bad → Eat Now → Feel Better (Temporarily)

When you feel a feeling (I know, groundbreaking), your brain goes, "Ugh. Gross. Let's not."

And it reaches into its bag of tricks — mostly built in childhood, reinforced by Netflix and capitalism — and pulls out the food card. Why?

Because it works.
Temporarily.

Eating does soothe. It releases dopamine. It blunts cortisol. It gives your nervous system the equivalent of a fluffy blanket and a quick lie down.

But then...
The original emotion is still there.
Now layered in guilt, bloating and an existential crisis about whether you should go keto.

Welcome to the emotional eating spiral — now featuring self-loathing and stretchy pants.

Feelings Aren't the Enemy (Even the Crappy Ones)

We live in a world that teaches us to avoid discomfort at all costs.

Sad? Swipe.

Anxious? Scroll.

Lonely? Order Uber Eats and pretend the delivery driver is your friend.

But feelings are like toddlers — the more you ignore them, the louder they scream.

They don't vanish. They just hide under the surface... until they bust out mid-meeting or during an ad for puppy rescue.

So here's the radical truth:

Feeling your feelings won't kill you.
Suppressing them, numbing them and eating them might not either... but it *sure as hell* won't help.

And this — right here — is the uncomfortable pivot point where real change happens.

Feel It to Free It (Yes, That Sounds Woo. No, I Don't Care.)

Let's try this:

Next time you feel the pull to emotionally eat — **pause.**

Yep, *her* again. The Pause. The Beyoncé of this book.

Instead of sprinting for the chocolate, stop for 10 seconds and ask:

"What am I actually feeling right now?"

Let it land. It might be messy. It might be vague.

But name it. Sit with it.
Cry if you need to.
Swear. Breathe. Journal. Yell at your indoor plant.

Just *don't run from it.*

Because every time you feel an emotion and don't run to the fridge, you're building emotional muscle. And eventually, it gets easier.

What To Do Instead (When You'd Rather Eat Than Feel)

Right — let's get practical. Here's your emotionally-savvy, BS-free toolkit for those snack-seeking stormy moments.

1. Ask: What's the Real Need?
Food's a stand-in. What's the *real* thing you're craving?
Connection? Rest? Peace? A break from your kids?

2. Self-Soothing, Not Self-Sabotage.
Make a list — a literal list — of non-food comforts.
Call a friend. Listen to a song that hits you in the chest. Take a walk. Wrap yourself in a blanket and pretend you're the main character in a moody indie film.

3. Don't Demonise the Food.
If you *do* eat emotionally, okay. Cool. You're human.
Just notice it. Be curious. Learn from it.
Then move the hell on.

4. Rewind Later.
After the storm passes, reflect. Not with judgement — with gentle investigation.
What triggered you?
What might help next time?

This isn't about "never eating emotionally again." That's not realistic.

It's about **breaking the cycle of reaction** — and stepping into *response*.

How? By pausing.

You're Not Weak — You're Wired. But You're Also Wise.

Let's close with this: emotional eating isn't a character flaw.

It's not laziness. It's not lack of willpower.
It's a strategy. A coping mechanism. A brain shortcut that once helped... and now maybe doesn't.

You don't need to bully yourself into behaviour change.
You need to *understand* yourself into it.

Because once you see the pattern — once you recognise that what you've been calling a "lack of control" is actually just a well-worn emotional path — you can step off it.

You can build new responses. You can meet your feelings with kindness. You can trust yourself to handle discomfort without crumbling into cookie crumbs.

You don't have to be perfect.

Just *aware*.

And pausing helps you do that.

Next up? Chapter 9: *The Inner Critic vs. The Inner Coach — Who's Really Running the Show?*

Because if you've got a voice in your head telling you you're a failure... it's time to fire her and hire someone a lot more helpful.

So let's crack on and meet the upgrade: your Inner Coach.

9

〜〜〜

The Inner Critic vs. The Inner Coach

Who's Really Running the Show?

*IN WHICH WE MEET THE TWO MAIN CHARAC-
TERS IN YOUR HEAD: THE ONE WHO KEEPS
YOU STUCK AND THE ONE WHO'S BEEN
GAGGED AND DUCT-TAPED IN THE CORNER,
BEGGING FOR HER MOMENT.*

You know that voice in your head?

The one that pipes up just as you open the fridge and says something delightful like, *"Well done, genius. I guess we're failing again today,"* or *"Go ahead, eat the muffin — because clearly THAT'S going to fix your life."*

Yeah. Her.

Meet **The Inner Critic**.

She's mean. She's dramatic. She's got the emotional range of a soap opera villain and the subtlety of a marching band in a library. And she's been narrating your food choices, body image and life decisions like she's auditioning for a part in *Mean Girls: The Inside Voice Edition*.

But here's the twist: she's not evil.
She's scared.
And kind of confused.
And tragically misinformed by decades of diet culture, toxic productivity and that time Prudence in Year 9 called you "chubby" in PE.

But we'll get to her therapy bill later.

Because there's *another* voice.
One that doesn't shout over you or shove guilt down your throat.

She's quieter.

Kinder.

Wiser.

The kind of voice that doesn't throw a tantrum when you eat carbs.

She doesn't judge.
She doesn't mock.
She doesn't suggest you swap your joy for a stick of celery and pass it off as "wellness."

She's not trying to shrink you.

She's trying to *guide* you.

Back to balance. Back to sanity. Back to *you*.

And when you give her even a sliver of airtime —
a pause, a breath, a second of not reacting —
she shows you the way through.

Not with control.
Not with chaos.
But with clarity.

She's **The Inner Coach.**
And my friend — *she* is the one we're here to unleash.

Two Voices, One Head — It's Basically Hamlet, But With Crumbs Down Your Shirt

Let's visualise this.

You walk into the kitchen.

Critic: *"Oh look, here we go again. Can't stick to anything, can you?"*

Coach: *"Hey love, rough day? What do you actually need right now?"*

Critic: *"Well, it's not a salad, clearly. Maybe try willpower for once in your life."*

Coach: *"You're tired. It's okay. Let's take a breath before we decide."*

See the difference?

The Critic attacks.
The Coach *supports.*
One shames you into submission. The other leads you with compassion.

And yet — who do we listen to most of the time?

That's right. The b*tch with the megaphone.

Why?
Because she's louder.
Because she's been rehearsing her script since 1997.
And because somewhere along the way, we mistook *bullying* for *motivation*.

Your Brain, On Scripts

Now for a little neuroscience — don't worry, I'll keep it sexy.

The Inner Critic is basically your brain's safety officer on steroids.

Her job? Keep you in the *known zone* — even if the known zone sucks. Even if it's filled with self-loathing, diet rules and shame spirals.

Because familiarity = safety to the brain.

She uses old scripts to keep you behaving in familiar ways. Stuff like:

- *"You always fail."*
- *"You're lazy."*
- *"You don't deserve to eat that."*

It's predictable. Safe. And absolute bollocks.

Meanwhile, the Inner Coach?
She operates from your **prefrontal cortex** — the CEO of the brain. She's calm. Considered. Big-picture thinking. She's the one who makes decisions based on your values and your goals, not your panic or your past.

She's basically your mental Beyoncé, but with a better understanding of blood sugar.

The trouble is: she only comes online when you *pause.*
You remember the Pause, right?

That moment of stillness before the fridge door swings open.
The breath before the biscuit.
The beat before you react.

That's her window.
But if you're rushing, judging or already elbow-deep in a bag of crisps, you won't hear her over the Critic's full-blown TED Talk on why you're the human embodiment of disappointment.

◈ Whose Voice Is That, Anyway?

Here's a curly question:

Is the voice in your head even *yours*?

Was it your mum?
Your Year 5 teacher?
The diet industry?
Oprah in 2003?

So many of our inner critics are just old voices we internalised and never questioned.

You don't pop out of the womb thinking, *"My thighs are offensive."*
You learn that crap.
Then it becomes automatic. And automation is powerful — until you *notice* it.

Because once you hear it... you can change it.

The Rewrite: From Self-Criticism to Self-Leadership

Now, I'm not saying you need to hold hands with your Inner Critic and sing Kumbaya under a full moon. (Although if that's your thing, you do you.)

I'm saying: **it's time to retrain your internal script.**

Step 1: **Catch the Critic.**
Notice her. Literally say, "Oh, there she is again."
This separates *you* from *her*. You are not that voice. You're the one *hearing* it.

Step 2: **Challenge the Crap.**
Ask, "Is that even true?"
Is it true you *always* fail? Or is it just that your brain loves a dramatic headline?

Step 3: **Coach It Up.**
What would your Inner Coach say instead?

Not toxic positivity. Not "You're perfect and everything is fine."
But *truthful kindness.*

- "You're struggling. That's okay. What do you need?"
- "You can reset. You don't need to punish yourself."
- "Your worth is not measured in carbs."

Keep these phrases somewhere visible. Tattoo them on your forehead backwards if necessary. (Kidding. Mostly.)

Reclaiming Your Mental Mic

Here's the deal:
You don't get rid of your Inner Critic by hating her. You quiet her by *choosing* someone else to lead.

You become the adult in the room.
The compassionate boss.
The calm in the chaos.

And every time you do that, even once, you carve a new neural pathway — a groove in your brain that says: *"Kindness is allowed here."*

Over time? That groove becomes a road.
Then a motorway.
Then a default setting.

And *that*, my friend, is how you change the game — not by silencing the Critic completely, but by pausing, noticing, then turning her down and turning yourself **up**.

Final Note From Your New Mental Narrator

This isn't about doing things perfectly.
It's about becoming *aware*.
It's about choosing who gets the mic.

You can't control every thought that pops up.
But you *can* choose which one you feed. Which one you follow.
Which one gets to influence your next bite, breath or brave decision.

And that's not woo-woo.
That's neuroplasticity, baby.

So next time the Critic pipes up mid-meal with her Greatest Hits Compilation of Shame and Regret, take a pause, nod politely and say:

*"Thanks for your input, Prudence.
But today, the Coach is driving."*

Next up? Chapter 10: Take In the Good — Rewiring a Brain That's Hooked on the Negative

Because your brain's basically a drama queen with a PhD in catastrophising — obsessing over that one mini choccy at 3:27pm like it's a war crime.

Time to teach it a new trick: noticing the good stuff... and actually letting it land.

Let's rewire this glorious mess, shall we?

10

❦

Take In the Good

Rewiring a Brain That's Hooked on the Negative

OR: HOW TO CONVINCE YOUR BRAIN THAT NOT EVERYTHING IS ON FIRE AND YOUR THIGHS AREN'T A NATIONAL EMERGENCY.

Right, here's a not-so-fun fact to nibble on before we get to the brain snacks:

Your brain is Velcro for bad stuff and Teflon for good.
Yup. The wet spaghetti mess between your ears is evolutionarily wired to notice everything terrible, alarming, mildly inconvenient or that might result in your death... including Beryl from Accounts making that face when you reach for another biscuit.

But - and this is important — **you are not your cavewoman brain**. You're just renting space inside it.

And if you've spent the last however-many-years absorbing diet culture, Instagram thinspo and random advice from people who treat "cheat day" like a moral compass — then congratulations!

You've likely got a brain that's learned to scan for danger in every cupcake and panic at the sight of a carb.

Which is exactly why we need to talk about *taking in the good.*

Because here's the scandal:
The *pause* we've been banging on about?
It doesn't just stop the autopilot.
It creates a *window.*
And in that little window, you get to choose: feed your brain something life-giving or let it munch on anxiety and shame with a side of self-loathing.

Let's break it down, shall we?

Negativity Bias — Your Brain's Junk Mail Filter Is Broken

Picture this. You have one average Tuesday.

- You eat a decent breakfast.
- You respond to 14 emails without telling anyone to shove it.
- You skip the biscuit tin.
- You remember your water bottle.
- You even make a salad for lunch with *actual vegetables.*

But then, at 3:27pm, you eat a mini chocolate bar.

And what does your brain do?

"WELL DONE, YOU ABSOLUTE FAILURE. THERE GOES EVERYTHING. MIGHT AS WELL ORDER A PIZZA AND WRITE OFF YOUR LIFE."

One slip and your brain's all dramatic, like Shakespeare on a blood sugar crash.

That's because your brain, in its natural prehistoric paranoia, thinks bad things are *more important*.
Survival, remember?

Back then it was:

- Sabre-toothed tiger? FOCUS!
- Delicious berries? Meh, we'll get to those.

Now it's:

- Muffin in the staff kitchen? DANGER. Don't eat it, or else!!
- Salad? Yawn. Maybe later.

But if we want to stop treating food like a battlefield, we have to retrain the brain to *notice what's going well*.

To *absorb* it.
To *dwell* on it — not like a creepy ex, but like a warm, reassuring blanket knitted by your nanna who always knew you were a legend.

The Science Bit — Grow the Good or Stay in the Cr*p

Neuropsychologist Donald Hebb — who really knew his stuff — inspired the now-iconic phrase:

"What fires together, wires together."

In other words: the more you focus on something — the more your brain physically changes to accommodate it.

If you constantly ruminate on your food fails, body flaws and internalised guilt over toast — your brain strengthens those neural networks like it's building a guilt-themed gym.

But *what if* — instead of galloping through your day like a caffeinated squirrel on a treadmill — you paused.

Just... paused.
Long enough to notice a flicker of joy, a glimmer of calm or even just a solid "meh" of neutrality?

Because when you do that — *ta-da!* — your brain, that weird little squishy computer between your ears, starts *rewiring* itself.
Like, genuinely.
Scientifically.
Neuroplasticity, baby.

It's like switching stations from "All Guilt, All the Time" to a smooth, low-fi frequency called *You're Doing Fine FM.*
No static. No shame. Just sweet, sweet sanity.

So... what's pleasure got to do with it?
Everything, Tina. Everything.

Here's the tragicomic routine most women star in (without auditioning):
You wake up and boom — it begins.
Tick boxes. Pack lunches. Answer emails.
Defuse emotional bombs disguised as toddlers.
You hustle like there's an invisible panel judging your performance (Spoiler: there isn't. They've gone home. They're eating cheese.)

And in this Olympic sprint of obligation, you miss the glitter.
The *confetti moments.*
Like...

- The sun warming your cheeks like a tiny celestial hug.
- A stranger holding the door like a background extra in a feel-good rom-com.
- Your dog looking at you like you're made of bacon and dreams.
- That one person who says "great job" and means it.

But do you stop to bask in it?
Do you let your heart throw a tiny party?

Nope.
You mutter "aww, nice," like a robot who's just seen its first rainbow — and return to your sacred scroll of to-dos.

And then... comes nightfall.
The second shift.
Family, dishes, spreadsheets, rogue socks... whatever your brand of chaos is.

And *finally* — in that 9:47pm moment when the world is quiet and you've officially run out of sh*t to do — you think:
"Pleasure. Now, please."

And your brain, starved and twitchy, goes full raccoon in a bin.
"CHOCOLATE!" it screams.
"WINE! CHIPS! THREE CHEESES MELTED INTO ONE GIANT CHEESE!"

Because you've had *no joy all day*.
You skipped the little hits, so now you're chasing the big ones.

And let's be clear — it's not because you're weak or greedy or broken.
It's because you're human. With a brain. That wants dopamine. Like... now.

But here's the real kicker:
If you don't sprinkle your day with pleasure, your brain will start to believe food is the only joy you've got.

Which is bollocks. But also, biology.

So what's the fix?
Pause.
Breathe.
Notice the micro-moments of magic — the little "ooooh"s before the "nom nom nom"s.

Because when you feed your soul tiny pleasures, your brain stops begging for giant ones.

And suddenly, food becomes just food again — not a consolation prize for surviving the day.

The 10 (ish)-Second Trick to Change Your Brain (For Real)

Here's a tiny, mighty practice.
I call it **Savour & Soak**.

Step 1: Notice something good.
Doesn't have to be profound. Could be:

- You put your phone down while eating.
- Someone smiled at you.
- Your tea was *just* the right temperature.
- You paused before inhaling your lunch.
- You said "no" to a second helping because you were actually full (not because you're being "good").

Step 2: Pause and stay with that good feeling for 10–20 seconds.
That's it.

Just *feel* it.
Let it land.
Let your nervous system *feel* the goodness.

Step 3: Let it grow.

Imagine the good feeling expanding — like sunlight in your chest.
You're embedding it into your brain.
This is the "rewiring" bit.

Because every time you savour these moments, your brain learns:
"Ahhh, this is safe. This is good. Let's come back here."

That's called **installing the good** — and it's what helps your brain learn
a new pattern. Not by force. But by repetition.

And when your brain's less wired for stress and deprivation, your cravings naturally soften.
You don't need to eat your way to joy — because joy's been sprinkled
through your whole day like glitter (the good kind).

But Caroline, I Hear You Cry, Isn't That Just Toxic Positivity?

Nope.

This isn't about *pretending* everything is fine while your life is
metaphorically on fire and you're trying to eat your way out with a
pack of Tim Tams.

This isn't delusion.
It's *attention.*
It's noticing what's *actually* there — not just the chaos, but the quiet
wins too.

The whole messy, magnificent, occasionally melted spectrum.

It's about saying:

- "Yes, that was a rough day — AND I made it through."
- "Yes, I ate more than I wanted — AND I paused before going back for more."
- "Yes, my jeans are snug — AND my body is still worthy of kindness."

It's not pretending.
It's perspective.

And it's a radical act when your brain is used to flogging you like a dodgy personal trainer with a six-week shred plan and unresolved issues with women.

The Bottom Line (Because You've Got Things to Do)

You're not going to outrun your inner critic with willpower.
You're not going to heal by hating yourself more.
You won't change your eating habits by shaming your way skinny.

But here's the actual magic trick:

You *can* change — Not by force, but by *noticing*.

One delicious, tiny pause at a time.

Because for years, you've been running the same unhelpful programme:
"I'm broken. I have no willpower. I'm just someone who can't."
Darling — it's dodgy software. Time for an update.

Let's start giving your brain *actual* evidence that you're not a disaster in activewear.
You're just human. Gloriously, gorgeously, chaotically human.
And guess what?

There are moments of calm. Of peace. Of neutrality.

Tiny sparks of "Oh... that felt kinda good."

And when you notice them — really *let them in* — your brain goes: *"Wait... is this... happiness without doughnuts?!"*

You start to realise: Food isn't the main event.

It's not the headliner.

It's the supporting act in the rich, messy, magnificent musical that is *your life.*

You're feeding your brain something new to chew on —

And it's tastier than guilt.

It's called satisfaction. It's called permission.

It's called being the kind of woman who can pause mid-craving and go, "Ooh, look at me — being all emotionally evolved and sh*t."

Go on.

Savour it.Soak it in.

Smirk smugly if you must.

You've earned it.

Next up?

Chapter 11: Scarcity Brain — Why You Panic Eat Like It's the Zombie Apocalypse.

Spoiler alert: The problem isn't you. It's diet culture with a bullhorn yelling *"Eat it now! You'll never have it again!"*

Let's unpack it, shall we?

11

Scarcity Brain

Why You Panic Eat Like It's the Zombie Apocalypse

Imagine this: You walk into your kitchen. You've just had dinner. You're not hungry. You even said, "I'm so full I could pop." But now you're pacing the pantry like a meerkat in a drought.

You spot the Tim Tams. There are two left.

Cue internal chaos:

"What if someone else eats them?"
"I'll just have one... but then there's only one left and I'll just think about it all night."
"Actually, I should just finish them so they're gone and I won't buy any more."

Next thing you know, you're knee-deep in crumbs and regret, muttering something about "starting again Monday."

Congratulations. You've just met your **Scarcity Brain** — the primitive part of your noodle that believes food is about to be outlawed and you're on a game show where only one survivor gets dessert.

Let's take a closer look, shall we?

The Evolutionary Blame Game

Scarcity Brain is not your fault. It's evolution's twisted joke.

See, your brain hasn't evolved much since the days when food was something you *foraged*, not UberEats-ed. Back then, if you stumbled across a fig tree or a fat juicy mammoth, you *ate the damn thing*. Because you didn't know when your next feed would be — it could be tomorrow or next Tuesday. So your brain developed a clever little hack called **urgent consumption**.

Fast-forward 100,000 years and you live in a world where you can get a double choc muffin delivered at 2am by a man named Gary in a Hyundai i30... but your brain still thinks you might starve.

Enter Scarcity Brain. It whispers:

"Eat it now. All of it. Before it's gone. Before someone else gets it. Before you change your mind and start being 'good' again."

It doesn't care that you've got a fridge full of ready-to-eat meals and a pantry that could feed a scout troop. Scarcity Brain isn't logical. It's emotional. It's dramatic.

It's basically a Kardashian having a meltdown in your skull.

Diets: Scarcity Brain's BFF

Now, if Scarcity Brain was just about biology, we could probably work with it.

But oh no, society had to go and slap some diet culture on top, didn't it?

Every time you've said, *"I'll just be good this week,"* or *"No more carbs from tomorrow,"* or *"This is my last hurrah"* — you've been reinforcing the idea that food is about to disappear.

So your brain, being the overachieving little survivalist that it is, reacts like you've announced an impending famine. It triggers panic. It amps up cravings. It convinces you that eating four muffins in one sitting is a *completely rational act of self-preservation.*

Scarcity Brain doesn't understand moderation. It understands now or never. Feast or famine. Zombie apocalypse or bust.

The 'F*ck It' Spiral

Let's talk about the star of this particular horror film: the *F*ck It Moment.*

You know the one. It usually arrives after a long day, when you've already had something you "shouldn't" and your brain decides, "Well, I've blown it now, might as well eat the entire continent of Europe."

Scarcity Brain LOVES this moment. It practically throws a party. Because now it has permission to feast *before restriction returns tomorrow.*

This, my friend, is the binge-restrict cycle — a psychological pendulum where you swing between control and chaos, all because your brain is reacting to *perceived* deprivation.

You're not greedy. You're *triggered.* There's a difference.

The Illusion of "Getting It Out of the House"

How many times have you eaten something just to "get rid of it"?

I hate to break it to you, but your stomach is not a bin. You're not "getting it out of the house," you're just moving it from cupboard to colon.

If the idea of throwing out food gives you hives, you're not alone. Many of us were raised on "waste not, want not" or "clean your plate" mantras. But let's be honest: inhaling stale cupcakes in the dark isn't saving starving children.

It's just feeding Scarcity Brain.

How to Outsmart the Apocalypse

Okay, so how do we disarm this dramatic little diva?

Here's your anti-zombie action plan:

1. Stop threatening famine

Every time you tell yourself a food is "bad," or that you can't be trusted around it or that you'll cut it out tomorrow, your brain hears *"scarcity incoming!"*
Instead, practise **food neutrality**. Pause, then say: "This is just food. I can have it if I want. Is this what I actually want right now?"

2. Stock your "scary" foods

I know — wild. But keeping the Tim Tams *in the house*, accessible and guilt-free, signals to your brain that food is *not* running out. At first, you may still overeat. That's okay. It's the brain testing the theory. But with time, the urgency fades.

3. Pause. (Obviously.)

Before you eat, take a hot second to breathe. Check in. Are you hungry? Emotional? Just afraid the zombies will get there first?

This isn't about saying no to food. It's about making space to choose — not react.

4. Reassure your brain

Literally. Say it out loud: *"There is enough. I can have more tomorrow. I am safe."*
Yes, it feels weird. But your primitive brain needs *repetition and reassurance*. It's like a toddler — give it certainty and a snack.

Final Thought: You're Not Broken — You're Brilliant

If you've panic-eaten like it's your last night on Earth, that doesn't make you a failure. It makes you **human**. A beautifully complex creature trying to survive in a world of diet rules and 3-for-1 family packs of Maltesers.

Scarcity Brain is just your brain doing its job — badly.

But now, you've got the pause. You've got awareness. And that makes you dangerous — in the best possible way.

So next time the zombie apocalypse hits and you find yourself reaching for the whole loaf of sourdough, just pause...
...and remember:

There's enough. You're enough. And tomorrow, the bakery will still be open.

Next up? *Chapter 12: The Pause in Real Life — Pausing When You'd Rather Not*

Where we dive into what *real-life* pausing actually looks like.

Spoiler alert: it's not Instagram-worthy. But it *is* powerful.

Because in those messy, middle-of-the-chaos moments, the pause is where your power lives.

12

⚜

The Pause in Real Life

Pausing When You'd Rather Not

Ah yes, *the pause.*
It sounds so peaceful, doesn't it? So elegant.
"Just take a breath," they say. *"Tune in. Get curious. Choose with awareness."*
Right.
Meanwhile, your brain is doing cartwheels. Your kid is tantruming over a banana that broke in half. The dog's eaten your AirPods. Work sent an email titled "Quick favour."
And your body?
Your body just wants couch, wine and something crunchy.

THIS, my friend, is when the pause gets real.

Because *this* isn't the version of pausing you see in mindfulness memes with sunset yoga and rose quartz vibes.
This is the messy, muttering-to-yourself, *"Don't scream at the cheese drawer"* kind of pause.

So let's talk about it. What pausing actually looks like when you *really, really* don't want to.

Step One: Accept That You're Going to Want to Punch This Chapter

Let's get one thing straight: pausing is *not* glamorous.

It's not some enlightened, glowy moment where you close your eyes, become one with the cosmos and whisper, *"Ah yes, I am aware of my triggers."*
No.
Real-life pausing is more like this:

You: "I'm not even hungry, but I'm eating this anyway."
Also you (in a whisper, holding a cracker): "Pause, you idiot. Just... pause."

Sometimes it's a breath. Sometimes it's a full-blown *internal wrestling match.*
And sometimes — let's be honest — you don't pause at all. You just bulldoze straight into the snacks and THEN go, *"Well that escalated quickly."*

That's okay. You're human. Not some emotionless carb-avoiding cyborg.

But Why Is It So Bloody Hard?

Because when your nervous system is lit up like a Christmas tree and your thoughts are racing like a caffeinated squirrel, asking your brain to pause feels like asking a Formula 1 driver to *just do a three-point turn real quick.*

Let's not forget, your stress-response system is ancient. It's not programmed for pause and reflection. It's programmed for *fight, flight or shove the Doritos down your throat while watching true crime.*

So no, in the heat of the moment, pausing doesn't feel natural.
It feels weird.
Like trying to meditate in a mosh pit.
Like attempting yoga while being chased by a bee.

And yet — that's where the magic is.

Real-Life Pausing, Exhibit A: The End-of-Day Spiral

It's 8:49pm.
You've given all your rational brain cells to other people. You're emotionally bankrupt. The wine's whispering sweet nothings. And you're staring into the fridge like it holds the meaning of life.

Here's the script your brain runs:

"I deserve this. I've earned it. I've been good. It's been a DAY."
"One glass. One snack. One little something to take the edge off."
"Screw it, I'll just start again tomorrow."

And hey, maybe you *do* want the wine and the snacks — that's totally fine.

But the pause is what gives you the *option* to decide.

It's the moment where you zoom out just long enough to ask:

"What am I really needing right now? Is it food... or is it comfort, connection, silence, a hug, a nap or an adult who doesn't need me to sign a permission slip?"

You don't need to get it perfect. You just need to *interrupt the autopilot.*

Even for 10 seconds.

Because those 10 seconds?

They're the gap where change sneaks in.

Real-Life Pausing, Exhibit B: The Scream-Snack Situation

You've just had an argument. You're vibrating with rage.
You stomp into the kitchen and open the cupboard with more force than necessary (poor innocent cupboard). Your hand is halfway to the chocolate when you remember:

"Pause, you dramatic wench. Pause."

This is what a real pause might look like here:

- You yell, "ARGH!" into a tea towel.
- You stomp outside and whisper, "What the actual hell," to the moon.
- You put your hand on your belly and check if it's shouting *"feed me"* or *"feel me."*
- You take one exaggerated breath that feels totally pointless — and yet, somehow, creates 1mm of space.

That's it.
Nothing Insta-worthy. Just a moment of *not-reacting.* A gap between the thing that happened... and what you do next.

That's where your power is. Not in the food choice — in the *pause before the food choice.*

Pausing Isn't a Diet Trick — It's a Rebellion

Diet culture has trained you to react like Pavlov's dog.
Feel stressed? Eat lettuce.

Feel fat? Eat nothing.
Feel sad? Eat everything.
Start again Monday.

Pausing breaks that loop.

It says, "Hang on. I'm not a puppet. I don't have to react on cue."
It's an act of rebellion.
A middle finger to autopilot.

It's you saying:

"Even if I still choose the food, I want to know *why* I'm choosing it.
I want to be awake at the wheel.
I want to be the one driving, not just along for the ride."

The Magic's in the Imperfect Pause

Here's what no one tells you:
The pause doesn't have to be beautiful to work.
It can be ugly, awkward, late, messy and still be *bloody brilliant.*

Even noticing *after* you've inhaled half a loaf of sourdough and three rogue Tim Tams is still part of the process.

"Wow, I was totally hijacked there."
"Interesting — I didn't even ask if I was hungry."
"Next time I want to try pausing before I start."

That *reflection* is a form of pausing too. It's like pressing rewind with curiosity instead of shame. And every time you do that, your brain gets better at spotting the patterns earlier.

Final Thought: The Pause Is a Practice

Not a perfection.
Not a performance.
A practice.

You'll mess it up. You'll forget. You'll resist.
And then, one day, you'll catch yourself mid-habit, mid-craving, mid-chaos... and go:

"Oh. There it is. The moment. The pause."

And you'll choose — maybe differently. Maybe not. But it'll be *you* choosing. Not zombie-you. Not Scarcity Brain. *You.*

So next time someone tells you to *"just breathe,"* and you want to hurl a couscous salad at their head — remember:
They're not wrong.
They're just wildly underestimating the badassery it takes to *actually* do it.

Up Next? *Chapter 13: Your Body's Signals — Missed Calls from Hunger & Fullness*

Your body's been calling. You've just had it on silent.

Let's decode those mixed messages and help you tune into your body's wisdom that's been there all along.

No more silent mode. No more voicemail. Just clear signals—and the confidence to trust them.

13

⁓⁓⁓

Your Body's Signals

Missed Calls from Hunger &
Fullness

(PLEASE LEAVE A MESSAGE AF-
TER THE BEEP)

You know that feeling when your phone's been on silent all day and suddenly you notice 14 missed calls, three from your mum, two from your dentist and one that may or may not be from a telemarketer who now thinks your name is "Hellooo?"
Yeah. That's basically what your body's been dealing with.

Because here's the deal: your body has been calling you. Repeatedly. Hunger? Fullness? They've both been ringing.
But between diet culture, the 4,000 tabs open in your brain and that one voice in your head constantly yelling, *"You shouldn't be hungry, you just ate an hour ago!"*, you've been sending those calls straight to voicemail. Possibly for years.

Now, before you start feeling guilty — *don't*.

This isn't a blame-fest. This is a *reunion*.

Like a cheesy Netflix drama where long-lost siblings find each other through a trail of awkward letters and DNA tests, this chapter is about finally reconnecting with your body's signals.

Not perfectly. Not instantly.

But with curiosity, kindness and the willingness to fumble through it like someone trying to fold a fitted sheet.

Can You Actually Hear Hunger?

Let's begin with hunger. The real kind. Not the "that ad showed me melted cheese and now I'm emotionally compromised" kind. I mean physical hunger. The body's gentle, primal way of saying, *"Hey mate, we could do with some fuel down here. Not urgent yet, just a heads-up."*

But here's the thing: most of us don't hear it until it's no longer gentle. It starts like a whisper — a soft stomach tug, a drop in focus, a subtle emptiness.

We ignore it. Because meetings. Or guilt. Or the lingering voice of a trainer who once told us hunger is weakness and we should just "push through." (Spoiler alert: that person was wrong and possibly hangry themselves.)

Eventually, that whisper becomes a shout. You're snapping at your partner, contemplating crimes against vending machines and questioning all your life choices — one rice cake at a time.

This is what I call *rage hunger*. You don't choose what to eat. The hunger chooses *you*. And it always seems to choose whatever's closest, crumbliest and capable of being inhaled in four bites or less.

So let's change that.

Let's unmute the signals. Let's take hunger off silent mode and learn to feel it before we're one Snickers away from becoming a tabloid head-line.

Signs You're Actually Hungry (Like, Physically Hungry):

- A gentle ache or empty feeling in your stomach
- Feeling light-headed, cranky or foggy
- Finding yourself thinking about food without emotional drama
- Your body feels "low battery," not "emergency red alert"
- Food sounds *good* — not like a coping mechanism, but a delicious idea

Notice none of those signs say "you *should* be hungry" or "you *haven't eaten in X hours*"?

That's because your body isn't a bloody spreadsheet. It's a responsive, intuitive, semi-magical organism that doesn't give a toss about your eating schedule.

Fullness — The Other Forgotten Signal

Now let's talk about fullness. Sweet, polite, utterly neglected fullness. Fullness is like that friend who gently taps your shoulder at a party to say it's time to go, but you're too busy doing tequila shots with your bad decisions to notice.

It's there. Quietly. Patiently.
Saying things like:
"Hey, that was nice."
"We're good now."
"Maybe take a breath and see how we feel?"

But noooo. We eat past fullness like it's an Olympic event. Especially if it's "healthy" food. Or it's free. Or the dinner rolls are so warm and

so crusty on the outside. So soft and squidgy on the inside.
Just like an armadillo.

And to be fair, we've been taught to override fullness. To finish our plate. To not waste food. To clean up even when we're stuffed like a sad Christmas turkey in a Tupperware of shame.

But what if we didn't?
What if we *paused*? Mid-meal. Just for a sec.
Not to calculate calories. Not to debate worthiness.
But to ask, *"How am I doing?"*

Like a quick check-in. A moment of body conversation.
Not *"Should I keep eating?"* (because that's often code for "Am I allowed?")
But a gentle, curious, *"What would feel good right now?"*

But What If You Can't Tell?

Totally normal.

If you've been ignoring your signals, overriding them or actively gaslighting them with 1200-calorie diets and intermittent fasting apps that beep at you like a hormonal Tamagotchi — it's going to take time.

At first, tuning into hunger and fullness might feel like listening for Morse code underwater during a drum solo. That's okay.

Your body hasn't stop talking. You just couldn't hear it over the noise of diet culture and Instagram wellness wankery.

Start small.

Pause *before* you eat. Ask, "Where am I on the hunger scale?"
Not to *earn* food. But to notice.

Pause *during* eating. Ask, "Am I still enjoying this?"

And — this is a wild one — pause *after*. Ask, "How did that feel?" (No shame. No scolding. Just data collection for your future self.)

Quick Hunger/Fullness Translation Guide:

- "I could eat" = Might be boredom. Might be actual hunger. Pause and ask.
- "I'm starving" = Probably missed earlier signals. It's okay. You're human.
- "I'm full but still eating" = Emotional need, habit or taste-chasing. Get curious.
- "I feel satisfied" = Huzzah! You've answered the call. Leave a 5-star review.

The Real Flex: Trust

This whole process is less about controlling what you eat and more about *trusting* that your body actually knows what it's doing.

Which is hard. Especially when you've been taught not to trust it. Thanks diet culture.

But the more you practice pausing, noticing, listening...

The more those missed calls become conversations.

And eventually? You'll be able to tell the difference between
"I'm hungry"
"I'm tired"
"I'm sad"
"I'm thirsty"
and
"I just saw a salted caramel brownie and my soul briefly left my body."

Final Thought

Your body isn't trying to sabotage you. It's not lazy or greedy or broken.
It's been calling.
It's always been calling.

You've just been *busy*.

Now...You're learning to pick up.

Even if it's awkward. Even if you drop the metaphorical phone a few times.
Every pause is you tuning back in.

And that, my friend, is a glorious, biscuit-crumb-covered revolution.

Next up? Chapter 14 — *Redefining Success.*

No rules. No rigid goals. Just noticing you're mid-biscuit and thinking, "Ah, the emotional-eating foxtrot."

We'll ditch the highlight reel and cheer for the pause—even if you still eat the damn thing.

Progress isn't polished or pretty. It's human.

14

Redefining Success

Or: "Yes, I Ate the Biscuit—But I Paused, Dammit!"

Most of us are so hardwired for all-or-nothing thinking that any-thing less than *flawless* feels like failure.

If you've ever said something like "I was doing so well until Friday happened," or "I totally blew it because I had a second helping of din-ner," then congratulations: you're in the right place, my friend.

Welcome to the black-and-white brain club. We meet on Mondays. There's tea. And maybe snacks. But only if we *pause* first.

Here's the inconvenient truth: success is not sexy. It's not a montage with dramatic music and green juices and someone sprinting up a hill at sunrise while looking mysteriously dewy.

Real success? It's gritty. It's weird. It's often invisible and mostly internal. It's pausing for two seconds before faceplanting into a muffin and going, *"Huh. I'm eating because I'm bored. Interesting."*

That's it. That's the win.

You noticed.
You *saw* yourself mid-pattern.
You woke up — even just for a flicker — before slipping back into autopilot.

That flicker? That's the gold. That's the bit that changes your life.

Not the absence of mistakes. Not a perfect streak of "good" food decisions.
But those tiny, awkward, blink-and-you'll-miss-it moments of *awareness.*

Let's put it this way: if your brain is like a freight train that's spent years barrelling down the same track (say, the *"Feel Emotion, Must Eat"* Express), then success isn't derailing the train overnight. It's sticking a bright yellow post-it note on the dashboard that says, *"Hey, is this the only option?"*

And maybe one day, eventually, you'll nudge the lever and try a new direction.

But the first success is *seeing the damn lever.*

The Myth of "Getting It Right"

There is no "right."

I hate to break it to you, but that pristine day where you eat nothing but quinoa, feel nothing but joy and meditate before every bite?

That day doesn't exist. Unless you've been kidnapped by a wellness cult and they've confiscated your phone. And even then, I give it 24 hours before you start fantasising about nachos and swearing at a wind chime.

Here's the truth: being human is gloriously inconsistent. You'll have days when you nail the pause, sit with your feelings like a Zen monk and walk away from the biscuit tin with the smug satisfaction of a self-actualised goddess. And then you'll have days when the only thing you manage to pause is the Netflix episode between mouthfuls.

Both are valid. Both are part of the process.
Success isn't about *always* choosing differently. It's about *remembering* you have a choice.

Let Me Be Blunt (Because Subtle Isn't My Style)

If you paused — even slightly — before devouring the snack, scrolling your ex's Instagram or launching into that third glass of wine with a side of existential dread... that's success.

Seriously.

You don't need to throw out all your coping strategies tomorrow and replace them with bootcamp, journalling and herbal tea. (Unless herbal tea is code for wine. In which case, carry on. No judgement.)

You just need to pause. Even badly.

Real Success Looks Like:

- Saying, "Ugh, I know I'm not hungry but I want it anyway" and eating the damn thing *without shame.*
- Catching yourself halfway through the packet and going, *"Well, that escalated quickly,"* instead of numbing out entirely.

- Pausing for ONE breath before an old habit — even if it didn't stop you.
- Saying, "This was hard today" and *not* using that as an excuse to write yourself off until Monday.

Can We Talk About Grace?

I know, it sounds like a nun or a fancy perfume, but *grace* is actually the superhero we've all been ignoring. Grace is what lets you mess up without throwing yourself under the metaphorical bus. Grace is the quiet voice that says, *"Yeah, that didn't go how you hoped. But you're still here. And that counts."*

Grace is *not* the same as letting yourself off the hook. It's not pretending everything's fine while white-knuckling a family-sized chocolate block.
It's pausing long enough to be honest — *without being a jerk to yourself.*

It's saying, "I didn't get it 'right,' but I showed up. I noticed. I tried."

That's the kind of success that actually lasts.

If You're Thinking Grace is the Same as Your Inner Coach, It's Not.

Grace and your inner coach are close cousins, but they're not the same person at the party. Think of it like this:

Grace is the vibe.
She's the energy that wraps around you when things go pear-shaped. She's the warm blanket, the deep exhale, the *"You're human, not a robot, love"* whisper after a rough day.

Grace lets you screw up and still see your worth.
She's not passive — she's radical in a quiet, firm, "try again tomorrow" kind of way.

Grace is what allows the pause.

She's the one who stops the spiral.

She's the reason you don't throw the whole day/week/month out the window because of one biscuit.

Your Inner Coach, on the other hand, is the voice inside you that responds *from* grace — not from shame.

She's the one who steps in *after* grace has softened the moment and says:

- "Okay, that happened. What do we want to do next?"
- "What did we learn?"
- "Let's not make this a drama. Let's make it a decision."

She's pragmatic. Supportive. Smart.

Not afraid to tell you the truth — but never in a way that makes you want to hide under the doona with a tub of ice cream and a side of guilt.

So, in short:

- **Grace** is the pause that gives you space to regroup.
- **Your Inner Coach** is the voice that helps you move forward from that pause.

One holds you.

The other helps you grow.

Together?

They're an unstoppable duo.

The Beyoncé and Lizzo of emotional regulation.

So What Now?

You keep showing up.

You keep pausing, even when it's awkward or late or you're halfway through a box of Shapes.

You keep choosing to notice rather than numb, to stay curious rather than cruel and to see every "off" moment as just another rep in your brain's emotional gym.

You *don't* wait for it to feel easy before you start.

You *don't* wait until you're "ready" or perfect or have all the right snacks.

You just keep practicing the pause — in all its messy, imperfect, biscuit-covered glory.

One Last Thought

Success isn't clean. It's not Instagrammable.

It's often invisible.

But it *is* happening — right now — every time you interrupt the loop, every time you hear your inner critic and pause before believing it, every time you *see* what you're doing, even if you do it anyway.

That's not failure. That's rewiring.

That's your brain changing.

That's a bloody miracle.

So stop measuring success by how long you stayed "on track" and start counting how many times you remembered you had a choice.

Because you do.

And you always have.

Even when you forget.

Even when you eat the biscuit.

Especially then.

So... you've redefined success, mid-biscuit.
You've paused in the chaos, dodged perfectionism and remembered that noticing is the win.

What now?

The epilogue. The encore. The philosophical burp at the end of the feast.

In the final chapter — *The Aftertaste: Living a Paused Life* — we zoom out.
Because this book? It was never just about what's on your plate.
It's about what's lurking behind the fridge door, running wild between your ears and bubbling under the surface of your busy, beautiful life.

It's the moment you realise: the pause was never just about food.
It was the door.
You were always the magic.

15

The Aftertaste — Living a Paused Life

So here we are.

The final chapter. The after-dinner mint of the whole experience. A little something to leave on your tongue as you shuffle back into real life — which, let's be honest, is already yelling, pinging, spilling and demanding to know what's for dinner. Again.

And here I am — your trusty narrator — waving a metaphorical champagne glass and whispering, *"You made it, you marvellous pausing creature, you."*

But before we part ways, let's step back and look at the big picture. Because *The Power of the Pause* was never *just* about food. That was just the door we crept in through.

Quietly. Holding snacks.

The real magic?
Is what pausing does to your entire freaking life.

A Brief Recap (for those of us with goldfish brains)

Let's rewind.

You started this book thinking, *"Maybe I eat on autopilot a bit."*
Next thing you know, you've wrestled your inner critic, stared down cravings like a boss, told diet culture to sod off and discovered that one tiny breath can be the difference between a meltdown and a breakthrough.

You've learned that:

- Pausing isn't passive. It's a power move.
- Emotional eating isn't weakness — it's a very creative attempt at survival.
- Scarcity brain is a total drama queen.
- You are *not* your cravings, your past or your pantry.
- And sometimes... you just want the bloody chocolate. And that's okay.

But more importantly, you've realised that when you pause — really pause — you become someone who chooses *on purpose*.

Not someone who reacts. Not someone who self-sabotages and then overanalyses it in bed at 2am. Not someone on a bloody hamster wheel of guilt, restriction and fridge-door therapy.

You become someone who responds.
With awareness. With kindness. With a twinkle in your eye and half a breadstick in your hand.

So... Now What?

Here's the part where I *could* leave you with a glowing list of "Top 10 Ways to Stay on Track Forever," complete with pastel fonts and words like "balance," "harmony" and "radiance."

But honestly? Real life is more like:

- You wake up late and step on a piece of Lego.
- You forget to defrost dinner (again).
- Someone cuts you off in traffic and you scream at them *in an accent* for some reason.
- You end up eating toast over the sink while Googling "Am I addicted to gluten?"

And that's why the pause matters so bloody much.

Because in those moments — the glorious, messy, un-Instagrammable ones — the pause isn't some cute habit.

It's your *lifeline.*

It's how you stop lashing out when you really just need a nap.
It's how you decide whether you need the biscuit, the bath or a boxing class.
It's how you pull yourself out of reactivity and land squarely in reality — where you can make a choice that actually serves you, not just soothes you for five minutes before the shame spiral starts.

The Pause Is Everywhere

This isn't just about food anymore.

This is about the conversation where you *don't* say the petty thing (even though it was SO GOOD and would've absolutely won the argument).

It's the email you don't send at 11:43pm when you're feeling emotionally flammable.

It's the "No" you give, with kindness and a side of confidence, because old-you would've said yes out of obligation and then resented everyone including the cat.

It's the moment where you pause before the scroll, the snack, the snap. Where you ask, *"Do I actually want this? Or do I just want to escape this moment?"*

It's how you become the version of yourself who's present, not panicked.
Intentional, not impulsive.
Connected, not just coping.

The pause is how you stop living life like it's a fire drill.

Nothing's Wrong with You. You're Just... Un-paused.

Here's something wild: you were never missing willpower.
You weren't "undisciplined" or "bad with food" or "emotionally weak."
You were just caught in *loops*.
Loops of reacting. Loops of rushing. Loops of not noticing what the hell was going on inside your own head.

Pausing breaks the loop.
It turns the whole system off, even if just for a second — enough to go, *"Hang on. Who's actually in charge here?"*

And surprise! **It's you**. It's always been you.
Underneath the panic, the patterns, the packet of chips — there you are.

Alive. Awake. A bit frazzled, yes, but sovereign as hell.

A Mini Manifesto: In Case You Need a Rally Cry for the Fridge Door

This is your reminder. Your reframe. Your poetic snack-time sermon.

I am not a robot.
I do not run on habit loops and marketing slogans.
I am not ruled by chocolate frogs, family feuds or calendar invites marked "Urgent."
I pause.
I feel.
I notice.
I decide.

I don't need to earn food, perform hunger or apologise for being human.
I can sit in discomfort without numbing it with cheese.
(Although occasionally I *will* numb it with cheese, because there are no rules.)

I trust my body.
I trust my cues.
I trust my messy, magnificent self to show up — again and again — even when I fall off the wagon, set it on fire and eat biscuits in the wreckage.

I am not here to live on autopilot.
I am here to be present.
To notice.
To pause.
And from that pause — to create a life that actually feels like mine.

Final Words (Before You Go Find Snacks)

Pausing won't make your life perfect.
But it will make it *yours*.

And that, dear reader, is better than perfect.
Because perfect is exhausting.

Perfect is fake.
Perfect never eats crackers in bed and whispers, *"I'll pause tomorrow."*

You do.
Because you're human.

So go forth. Live a paused life. Laugh often. Swear occasionally.
And when in doubt, breathe like you mean it.

Not because someone on a yoga mat told you to.

But because somewhere deep inside you, you *know*:

You're not here to react.
You're here to respond.
With grace. With guts.
And sometimes... with snacks.

THE END.

(Or maybe... just the beginning.)

Bonus Section

Frequently Asked Questions That Are None of Anyone's Business, But Here We Are

Q: Will this make me lose weight?
A: Maybe. Maybe not. Will it make you lose the icky mental weight of obsessing about food 24/7? Probably.
Will it help you stop treating your body like a malfunctioning robot that needs constant control and correction? Absolutely.
Also, your worth was never meant to be measured in kilograms. Or followers. Or the number of almonds you eat per sitting.

Q: But what if I forget to pause and end up face-down in a box of Tim Tams?
A: Welcome to the club, sweet pea. We have T-shirts. And crumbs.
This isn't about being perfect. It's about learning to say, "Huh, that happened," instead of, "I suck at life."
Try again. Pause again. Chocolate doesn't hold grudges and neither should you.

Q: Is this just intuitive eating with jazz hands?
A: Pretty much, yeah. But without the food moralising or the need to start a Pinterest board called Nourish.
It's tuning in without tuning out joy. It's science and common sense

with a sprinkling of irreverence and a strong cup of "bugger off, diet culture."

Q: So... what do I eat?
A: Whatever your body asks for in a tone that's not shrieking from the depths of emotional despair.
Some days that's kale. Some days it's lasagna. Some days it's a crisp apple.
And occasionally, it's wine and a wedge of brie the size of your face.
You're a grown woman. Trust yourself.

Q: Is it too late for me?
A: Darling, if you're still breathing and capable of chewing (or blending), it is never too late.
You can unlearn the madness. You can come home to yourself.
Start now. Start messy. Start with lunch.

One Final Pause

Right now, take a deep breath.
No, seriously. Inhale. Exhale. That's the good stuff.
You just gave your nervous system a tiny hug.

And that, my friend, is the work.
Not willpower. Not punishment.
Just presence. Just practice. Just you, showing up for yourself again and again until it feels like home.

Now go forth and eat like a gloriously free, occasionally chaotic, deliciously intuitive human being.

Pause often. Laugh much.

And never trust a diet that tells you to cut out carbs or joy.

Love from me — and your whispering body.

A Soundtrack to Pause By

aka "Tunes to Drown Out Diet Culture and Reclaim Your Sanity in 3–5 Mins or Less"

Because sometimes the difference between "I'll pause and breathe" and "I just shouted at a biscuit" is a bloody good song.

Here's a little sonic first-aid kit for your nervous system — no pan flutes or whale sounds unless you're into that sort of thing (in which case: flutes away, my love).

1. "Weightless" – Marconi Union

Scientifically proven to slow your heart rate and reduce anxiety. Like being hugged by a cloud wearing a lab coat.

2. "Dog Days Are Over" – Florence + The Machine

For when you remember you're not broken — you're just blooming. Loudly. With tambourines.

3. "Just Breathe" – Pearl Jam

A gentle, grungy reminder that even grizzly rock dudes pause and reflect.

4. "Lovely Day" – Bill Withers

If you need a musical pep talk that feels like sunshine in audio form. Use liberally.

5. "Shake It Out" – Florence again (because obviously)

Best played while dramatically pretending you're releasing shame from your shoulders. Bonus points for interpretive dancing in the kitchen.

6. "You've Got the Love" – Candi Staton / Florence (pick your fighter)

Play when you need to remember you've already got what you need inside you.
(Spoiler: It's not kale. It's self-trust.)

7. "This Is Me" – Keala Settle (from The Greatest Showman)

Because screw fitting in. You're showing up. Scars, hunger, cravings and all.

8. "Sweet Disposition" – The Temper Trap

For slow walks, reflective sighs or that moment before you decide not to eat your feelings but instead feel your feelings (ugh, I know).

9. "Human" – Rag'n'Bone Man

Because you are not a monk. You're not a machine. You're human — beautifully fallible and occasionally snacky.

10. "Tubthumping" – Chumbawamba

("I get knocked down... but I get up again...")
An anthem for every "oops, I ate my feelings again" night. Hit play, brush off the crumbs, carry on.

Pro tip: Make your own "Pause Playlist" — fill it with songs that calm your chaos, make you grin or remind you that you are a whole damn miracle. Stick it on when the urge to mindlessly munch hits and dance, breathe or simply be instead.

Because pausing isn't just about silence.
It's about tuning in.
And baby, your frequency is *fabulous*.

Tools to Keep Beside the Cheese Drawer

aka "Your Emergency Kit for When You're About to Emotionally Eat a Wheel of Camembert"

Because let's be honest: the cheese drawer isn't just where we store dairy — it's where we go when we're bored, anxious or one passive-aggressive email away from a full-blown existential crisis.

So, next to the brie and the Babybels, keep a few of these cheeky tools on standby — to pause, breathe and maybe not eat your feelings (unless they taste like cheddar, in which case... be gentle with yourself).

1. Sticky Notes with Sassy Questions

Write some soul-interrupting gems like:

- "Hungry... or hiding?"
- "Will cheese fix this... or just distract me?"
- "Would a cuddle do instead?"

Slap them right on the inside of the drawer, so they sass you gently at your most vulnerable.

2. A "Pause Button" Object

Could be a small stone, a coin or that weird souvenir magnet from Byron Bay.
Touch it before you grab the cheese — let it remind you to breathe, check in and decide on purpose what comes next.
Like a fidget spinner for your prefrontal cortex.

3. A List Called "Other Ways to Self-Sooth That Aren't Gouda"

Have it right there, laminated if you're feeling fancy.
Examples:

- Walk around the block like a moody poet
- Blast one of your "pause" playlist songs
- Cuddle your pet/partner/pillow
- Scribble in your journal like you're the misunderstood heroine of your own Netflix special
- Nap. You probably just need a nap.

4. Mini Notebook for Brain Dumping

Because half the time, your brain is just full. Write the rant, don't eat the rage.
Scribble down what you're feeling in that moment.
Name the emotion. Curse creatively. Doodle an angry cheese if you must.

5. A Tea Bag That Smells Like Safety

Keep a calming tea blend nearby — peppermint, chamomile or something woo-woo with lavender and dreams in it.
Make a cup instead of making out with the camembert. Sip. Breathe. Repeat.

6. A Mirror (Yes, Really)

Because sometimes, seeing your own face mid-craving is enough to spark a pause.
Not in a shaming way — in a oh hi, love kind of way.
Use it to ask yourself out loud, "What do I really need right now?"

7. An Index Card That Says This:

"Hey lovely. It's okay to want cheese.
But before you bite, just check in.
Are you hungry or just human?
Either way — I love you.
Sincerely, Future You."

Think of this drawer not as a danger zone, but as a sacred pause portal.
A moment of "hang on a sec" before the autopilot munch begins.
It's not about banning the cheese.
It's about building the skill to ask: is this what I actually need right now?

And if the answer is yes?
Slice, plate, savour.
And don't you dare feel guilty about it.

Acknowledgements

*Because apparently, writing a book isn't
a solo sport. Who knew?*

To every woman who's ever found herself elbow-deep in a bag of chips thinking, *"What the actual hell just happened?"* — this book is for you. You are not alone. You are not fundamentally flawed. You are simply human, hormonal and possibly sleep-deprived. I see you. I *am* you. And I promise, you're doing better than you think.

To my clients — the glorious, honest, whip-smart women who have cried, laughed, raged and eaten their way through this work with me — thank you for trusting me with your stories, your stuckness and your snack drawers. You are the reason this book exists and every page has a bit of your brilliance in it.

To the brilliant minds whose work has shaped my own (even if I took your research and made it sound like stand-up comedy): thank you for giving me the science to back up my sass.

To my gorgeous husband who fed me, hugged me or at the very least didn't ask what I was doing when I was staring into space during a "creative pause" (read: procrastinating) — I love you and your patience. Also, yes, I ate the last of the Fromage d'Affinois. No regrets.

To the doubters, the diet peddlers and the voice in my own head that occasionally whispered, *"Who do you think you are to write this?"* —

thank you for giving me the opportunity to pause, flip you the mental bird and keep going anyway.

To snacks: You were there for the free-flowing days, the verbally constipated days and the "I'm just going to write one more paragraph" days that turned into 11pm carb binges. Without you, this book would be thinner, but so would I — and that's not the goal.

And finally, to you, dear reader — for picking up this book, for staying with it (even through the weird bits) and for being open to changing how you see yourself and your relationship with food, feelings and the fast-paced world we live in. If you walk away from this book with one new pause, one less panic and a little more peace in your day — then I'm bloody proud of both of us.

You've got this.

Now go out there and pause like your life depends on it. (Because sometimes, it kind of does.)

With love, mischief and a very large cup of tea (yes, that is code for wine),

Caroline

xx

About the Author

AKA: Who wrote this thing and why should you care?

Caroline Trickey is a dietitian, eating psychology coach and self-confessed ex-cereal-straight-from-the-box eater. She helps women break up with food rules, ditch the guilt and finally find their way back to eating like a sane human again — with real food and a whole lot of "hell yes" at mealtimes.

With over 20 years in the health world (and several more spent personally testing the limits of emotional eating), Caroline knows a thing or two about what actually helps people change — and spoiler: it's not another 12-week shred or green smoothie challenge. It's learning how to *pause* — in the middle of cravings, chaos, criticism and cookies — and choose something different.

She's the creator of the *Perfect Gauge Process*, the *Urge Surfing* app, the *Veggie-licious cookbook* and several other delightfully useful things with names that make people go, "Ooh, that sounds clever." But mostly, she's just passionate about helping women feel at home in their bodies and at peace with what's on their plate.

When she's not helping clients out of food jail or writing books with dramatic titles, she can be found drinking tea, avoiding laundry or practising the sacred art of the imperfect pause.

Follow her work, learn more or download some free goodies at: **www.carolinetrickey.com**

www.ingramcontent.com/pod-product-compliance
Lightning Source LLC
Chambersburg PA
CBHW062145020426

42334CB00020B/2514